Overcoming Binge Eating

A Comprehensive Guide to Symptoms,
Causes and Treatment of Your
Overeating Disorder

Edward Standmore

ISBN-10: 1535392339
ISBN-13: 978-1535392334

DEDICATION

Anyone who has tried and failed to beat binge eating.
Anyone who has failed to try to beat binge eating.

CONTENTS

ACKNOWLEDGMENTS

Thank you to the following individuals and organizations who without their contributions and support this book would not have been written:

J R. Coffey, Ellen L. and L. Wilkinson for great contributions to writing and editing.
Shutterstock for the distinctive cover image.
V. Charlie for the cover artwork.

Edward Standmore

LEGAL NOTES

Edward Standmore

INTRODUCTION

Why Should You Be Interested?

This book will take you on a comprehensive binge eating journey. You will understand medical history, mainstream conjecture, internal and external triggers, probable root causes and emotional stressors.

Take your first step in overcoming binge eating today.

What Will You Get From This Book?

Thankfully, there are endless resources available now that can help you achieve freedom from the enslavement of food. People are starting to recognize binge eating as an eating disorder and are moving towards solutions that will help them regain control of their eating habits. They want to bring change to their unhealthy lifestyle and are willing to learn where to start.

This book will outline everything there is to know about binge eating and how to bring healthy changes to overcome this eating disorder. You will be able to find a practical guide with many strategies to break the binge-purge cycle that shapes Bulimia Nervosa.

When a person suffers from an eating disorder, the food they eat fails to nourish their body. Instead, the food is used to handle feelings of distress. Eating to manage emotional or psychological needs is also known as emotional eating. People who binge eat use food to put their emotions at ease. It is something they find comfort in to soothe themselves, regulate their moods, and basically use it as a coping mechanism to manage feelings they are unable to handle.

Many people use food to settle emotional distress, but some people go overboard. They may either control their eating to manage upsetting feelings or to distract their emotional being. Others start to eat out of control as a means to overcome their feelings of distress. This becomes a huge problem because as this eating behavior turns into a habit, the person loses their sense of control when it comes to food.

Overcoming an eating disorder requires the person to pay attention to their physical, as well as their psychological well-being. Programs that treat eating disorders mostly focus on diet and this is why such programs remain ineffective for the long run. To truly overcome an eating disorder, it is important for the person to face their feelings of distress that have been the main cause behind the eating behavior.

One of the main risk factors that are often found common across all eating disorders is low self-esteem. Developing self-esteem isn't only important for overcoming eating disorders but it is also important for recovery. Returning back to good health requires you to closely reflect upon everything that causes you stress and coming up with solutions to eliminate these triggers. A firm decision has to be made on your part to make choices that reduce these daily stressors.

Recognizing the fact that we have a choice to be healthy is the first step to start making healthy changes. When people suffering from eating disorders have all the help they need, they get the necessary motivation to start the recovery process by themselves without the need of professionals.

This book is a self-help guide that is designed to become a practical tool to help people overcome their binge eating behaviors. You will be able to get better insight into what's actually causing you to binge eat. The purpose of this book is to provide empowerment to healthy choices that will help bring positive changes.

By the end of this guide, you will have a better understanding of how your thoughts, emotions, and behaviors are connected together and how they affect each other. With this understanding, you will be able to take better control of your eating habits and essentially your entire life. This book can easily be used along with the help that you receive from your healthcare professional, though it is not intended to replace a medical assessment.

It is also not to be used as an alternative to professional help and neither does it offer solutions that will work overnight. Overcoming eating disorders and recovering to a healthier you will take time and effort.

Struggling with an eating disorder will take up a lot of emotional, mental and physical energy. In order to overcome binge eating disorder, you need to learn how to channel these energies in a way that will allow you to become a better version of yourself so you can finally start enjoying life to the fullest.

CHAPTER 1: WHAT IS BINGE EATING?

A Brief History of Binge Eating

Before the mid-1990s, "binge-eating" was not considered a separate eating disorder by the psychological community, but a co-current disorder associated with bulimia nervosa, one of two eating disorders recognized by the DSM-IV-TR (Diagnostic and Statistical Manual of Mental Disorders), along with anorexia nervosa. Medical doctors, unclear as to what they were dealing with, typically prescribed weight-loss pills or antidepressants (like Prozac), while psychologists used cognitive-behavioral therapy directed at changing how sufferers responded to "cravings." Meanwhile, support groups like Overeaters Anonymous promoted their standard "twelve-step program" as a viable treatment--with very limited success.

Finally introduced as a provisional (potential new) disorder deserving further study by the American Psychiatric Association in 1994, binge-eating disorder (BED) was initially categorized under ENOS (Eating Disorders Not Otherwise Specified) until shown to be significantly different in nature from bulimia nervosa or anorexia nervosa. Ultimately deemed a full-fledged psychological eating disorder deserving the investment of scientific resources, BED was included in the updated 2013 DSM-5—both validating those suffering this debilitating disease and prompting healthcare professions to begin serious scientific investigation.

People who suffer from binge eating disorder eat abnormally large portions. There are also physical and psychological implications for people who binge on food. They start having strong concerns about their weight and eating habits and many find themselves on a fast track to obesity, which then brings its own health concerns.

According to the American Psychiatric Association (APA), Binge Eating Disorder is defined as:

"Recurring episodes of eating significantly more food in a short period of time than most people would eat under similar circumstances, with episodes marked by feelings of lack of control. Someone with Binge Eating Disorder may eat too quickly, even when he or she is not hungry. The person may have feelings of guilt, embarrassment, or disgust and may binge eat alone to hide the behavior. This disorder is associated with marked distress and occurs, on average, at least once a week over three months."

It has only been in the last few years that a concerted effort has been made by the medical and psychological communities to recognize, understand, and develop applicable treatment. In that brief time, however, considerable insight has been gained into this potentially life-threatening illness. Insight into the symptoms, causes, and treatment of this all-too-common eating disorder.

Am I A Binge Eater?

By definition, "binge-eating" is described as eating an amount of food that is excessively larger than what most people would eat within a given period of time (generally, any two-hour period) under similar circumstances. And while this definition would seem to apply to many individuals at various times under various conditions (Thanksgiving dinners, for example), binge-eaters report a distinct sense of loss of control regarding food (feeling they lack the willpower to stop eating or control what or how much they eat) and experience at least three of the following five abnormal behaviors:

1. Eating much more rapidly than normal.
2. Eating until feeling uncomfortably full.
3. Eating large amounts of food when not physically hungry.
4. Eating alone to hide feelings of embarrassment at how much is eaten.
5. Feeling disgusted, depressed, or overwhelmingly guilty after eating.

Additionally, binge-eating is recurrent; occurring (on average) at least once a week for three consecutive months. Thus, the physical, psychological, and cyclical components that distinguish binge-eating, effectively separate it from the occasional "over-eating" and should not be confused.

Impact of Binge Eating

Of course, a lot of people may fit the above criteria and still not qualify as a binge eater, though the patterns and emotional states are quite common amongst people suffering from the eating disorder.

The food eaten by the person is often highly calorific. Most of the time, the flavor of the food is disregarded and food is merely eaten in large quantities in a short amount of time. In a Binge Eating Disorder, there is absolutely no purging, where the person attempts to prevent weight gain. The final impact is a significant weight gain and feelings of disgust with oneself.

Some binge eaters find themselves stuck in a cycle

where they diet, binge, self-criminate, and self–loath. A lot of time binge eating is quite subjective, where the person didn't plan on overeating but eventually did when the food was placed in front of them. The eating disorder leaves the person as if they are out of control and they cannot cope without bingeing.

Stages of Bingeing

Binges happen in four steps:

1. First is the tension build-up where the person feels anxious and bothered, without actually knowing why they feel this way.
2. Then comes the tension release where the person starts to relax as they binge eat. As they eat, they are able to let go of all their uncomfortable feelings, though this relief is short-lived.
3. Then comes the post-binge where the person starts to feel uncomfortable due to overeating. The symptoms include bloating, exhaustion, headaches, nausea, diarrhea and general lethargy.
4. Lastly, the person makes renewed promises for change. They may not eat anything at all for the next few hours or even go on a strict diet. Soon enough, the person goes back to stage one.

Most individuals suffering binge-eating disorder describe the mental and emotional agony that follows a binge as far more agonizing than the physical side-effects of the food they consume. And unlike those suffering bulimia nervosa (who often suffer binge-eating disorder as well), those with binge-eating disorder symptoms typically do not purge their food, fast, or exercise excessively to compensate for binges. Additionally, those individuals tend to diet more often, enroll in weight-control programs (often compulsively, one after another), and have a history of family obesity.

The Emotional Component of Binge-Eating

While there are a number of emotional components that come into play for binge-eaters, one common element that appears to characterize most sufferers is what psychologists describe as an "unconscious desire to escape from self-awareness." This means that essentially, they eat excessive amounts of food in a very short period of time to free themselves from their own critical eye. Patient profiling has shown that most binge-eaters suffer from unreasonably high personal standards and expectations— and are hypersensitive to what they perceive as the impossible demands of others. Accordingly, when such individuals find themselves unable to live up to high standards and expectations, they develop a negative view of themselves (about their looks and abilities), becoming overly concerned at how they are perceived by others. This hyper-awareness is typically accompanied by emotional distress (anxiety, depression, desperation—even suicidal thoughts) which they attempt to escape by focusing on their immediate environment, avoiding long term, purposeful thought. This narrowing of focus effectively circumvents normal sensibilities about eating, fostering an uncritical acceptance of irrational thought and behavior. Psychologists view this "escape model" of behavior as fundamental to most binge-eating scenarios.

Statistically-speaking, nearly 50 percent of all binge-eaters first try dieting to alleviate their unflattering view of themselves before turning to bingeing, representing 33 percent of those considered more "psychologically disturbed" than those who use straight-forward dieting (rather than bingeing) to regulate mood and self-image. Considered an "expressive disorder," binge-eating is an outward expression of deeper psychological problems. And while the word "craving" is often applied to this condition in pop literature, it should be understood that technically speaking, cravings involve euphoric and withdrawal elements not necessarily part of the binge-eating scenario (notwithstanding the 33 percent of individuals who binge to alleviate "bad moods"). Likewise, the application of the term "addiction" to binge-eating is both misleading and not within accepted mainstream psychological definition of what constitutes addiction. Although similar, there is a distinct and a significant difference.

Why Binge-Eating "Disorder"?

As even non-professionals eventually come to notice, mental and physical illnesses are categorized by various qualifiers among members of the healthcare professions, such as "disease" (i.e., Lyme disease), "condition" (i.e., psychological condition), and "syndrome" (i.e., toxic-shock syndrome), but few laymen understand the distinctions. Nonetheless, it is quite important to understand how this categorization pertains to this eating "disorder," as it brings clarification to how science views this illness, and how treatment is meant to affect it.

Despite the many physical aspects associated with BED (physical comorbidities), binge-eating disorder is regarded as a psychological rather than physical ailment (an aberrant social behavior), best managed by psychological therapy. That is not to say that medical doctors and other therapeutic practitioners cannot be helpful in alleviating many of the symptoms associated with binge-eating disorder, only that such approaches treat the symptoms, not the source(s) of the problem. Thus the first step to understanding binge-eating disorder is to acknowledge that you are dealing with a serious psychological issue—that manifests physically.

The question that now arises is: Who is most affected by this "disorder"?

CHAPTER 2: WHO IS MOST AFFECTED BY BINGE EATING?

By the Numbers

Statistically, binge-eating disorder (BED) effects an estimated 3.5 percent of American woman and 2 percent of American men over the age of 18 (as of 2010). That's one-in-thirty-five! In terms of hard, cold numbers, this translates to more than 5.25 million adult women and 3 million adult men suffering this debilitating disorder. According to research assembled by the National Institute of Mental Health (NIMH):

"[BED] should be considered a public health concern because symptoms of the illness appear to be more prevalent than other eating disorders [bulimia and anorexia], and it is strongly associated with obesity."

Following the 2007 Harvard Study that prompted Marc Lerro, executive director of the Eating Disorders Coalition (EDC) to announce in Forbes magazine:

"This [study] is a wake-up call for the federal government to do

more, like counting the number of people who die each year due to an eating disorder . . . and funding research to determine what is effective in treating eating disorders."

Since that statement, binge-eating disorder has become the #1 most common eating disorder, surpassing both bulimia nervosa and anorexia nervosa in incidence. But the numbers many find most disturbing are those pertaining to American children and youth.

According to the Center for Disease Control and Prevention, the percentage of obese children between the ages of 6–11 in the United States increased from 7 percent in 1980 to nearly 18 percent as of 2012. Similarly, the percentage of obese adolescents between the ages of 12–19 increased from 5 percent to nearly 21 percent over the same period.

Accordingly, as of 2012, more than one third of all American children and adolescents were classified as overweight or obese—with binge-eating one of the most pernicious conditions facing teens today. This spiraling issue is further complicated by conflicting cultural perspectives as to what is normal today—the media promoting ultra-thin physiques as healthy, while various ethnic groups promote well-rounded "BBW" body-types as sexually desirable. Meanwhile, unhealthy eating patterns are established among children and youth that ultimately interfere with normal physical and emotional development, and require professional intervention to correct..

CHAPTER 3: WHO IS THE BINGE EATER?

Mainstream Thoughts on Binge Eating

There is not one common mainstream reason that causes the binge eating disorder. The media usually mention a collection of factors, including psychological, physical, sociocultural, and familial factors. Of course, the standard mainstream factors are thought to differ from person to person.

To understand the commonly recognized underlying reasons behind binge-eating disorder (BED), it's thought that it's important to look at factors that make a person vulnerable. There could be predisposing factors, which develop the disorder and then there are precipitating factors that trigger the disorder once it has been established.

Predisposing factors revolve around psychological issues, such as low self-esteem, poor body image, depression, anger, anxiety, loneliness, lack of control over life, perfectionist tendencies, and difficulty in expressing emotions. It may also be in relation to sociocultural factors, such as narrow definition of beauty, weights, and shapes. Lastly, it could also be familial factors, such as genetics, disharmony within family, traumatic experiences or loss of a close one.

Precipitating factors revolve around the person's diet. When the person goes into starvation mode out of guilt, they get even stronger cravings for food because they are lacking nutrition, which eventually increases their loss of control over food portions. It could also be stress related where the person uses food as a coping mechanism to handle self-doubt or anxiety. Lastly, theories are also based around social pressure, such as being teased about appearance or weight.

Now. What does the research suggest?.

Cause-and-Effect Consensus

Among several highly-considered cause-and-effect theories supported today is the idea that binge-eating disorder (BED) is most often caused by environmental factors and/or traumatic events.

One prominent study indicates that women suffering BED categorically experience more adverse life events in the year prior to the onset of the symptoms of the disorder, and that binge-eating disorder is directly associated with how frequently negative events occur.

Additionally, research has established that individuals who suffer binge-eating disorder are more likely to have experienced physical abuse, mental abuse, and/or body criticism than their healthy counterparts.

Other so-called "risk factors" may include incidence of childhood obesity, long-term criticism of weight from friends or family, low self-esteem, depression, and incidence of physical, mental, or sexual abuse during childhood. A relationship between dietary restraint and the frequency of binge-eating behavior has also been shown in some studies.

While binge-eaters are often thought to lack self-control (and thus, the reason they can't stop eating), the root of such behavior may be linked to rigid dieting practices--strict dieting and binge-eating part of a vicious cycle of behavior.

A Ground-Level Portrait

While statistics may help spotlight the seriousness of binge-eating disorder (BED), at ground level, a much more specific portrait emerges.

In the clinical setting, a number of factors come into play not reflected in numbers alone. For example, cultural differences regarding what is considered "over-weight" or "obese" ultimately mean that most individuals who seek professional treatment for binge-eating are White females. This is not to suggest that men or other ethnic groups do not suffer this potentially life-threatening illness, only that men (of any ethnic group, any age) seek help for binge-eating and other eating disorders far less often, and that non-Whites less-often consider their eating habits a problem.

Additionally, although American youth represent the fastest-growing obese demographic in the world, the psychological component of over-eating is rarely recognized for the first few years of this behavior (the common belief being that all teens—especially boys— require more calories to grow and that junk-food bingeing is the normal way to get them), meaning few teenage girls know to seek professional help before the pattern is well embedded. This, coupled with the natural decline in attention to body-image after age 55, means that the typical patient seeking professional help for binge-eating disorder is a White woman between the ages of 20 and 50. And no matter the age, the scenario they describe is always the same:

"I need help! I try to control myself but I just can't! I can't eat a

few potato chips—I have to eat the whole bag! I can't stop at one or two donuts, if I buy a dozen—I have to eat all twelve! Last night—even knowing I was coming here—I sat down in front of the tube and ate a whole quart of ice cream—then went back for a second and scarfed that down, too! I know it's wrong, but I just can't control myself! Once I start eating, I just can't stop! I love food! I know it's shameful, but I do love food!"

And while this scenario echoes loudly in countless psychologists' and therapists' offices across the country every day, the goal for therapist and patient becomes much more elusive when the darker details of their binge-eating habits come to light: 2a.m. excursions to the local convenience store to buy arm-loads of junk-food to be consumed in the front seat of the car, behind the building. Secret food stockpiles placed strategically around the house—visited, inventoried, and upgraded with almost fanatical dedication. Sneaking off to near-by towns to indulge in all-you-can-eat buffets—away from friends and relatives who could witness the shameful behavior.

And every binge is different. One day it's sweets, one day it's pasta. One day it's salty snacks, the next greasy foods. And if they can't get potato chips—they'll settle for chicken-in-a-bucket. Can't get donuts—they'll settle for a giant tub of potato salad. No ice cream—no problem—a dozen king-size chocolate bars will do! And even after a bucket of chicken, tub of potato salad, and a dozen candy bars (with stomach bulging and breathing labored) they may contemplate driving to the nearest fast-food joint for something slathered in melted cheese. This is the binge-eater: Insatiable. Out of control. Sad and angry inside.

But, what sets-off the binge-eating habit? Is there a root cause?

CHAPTER 4: WHAT'S BEHIND THE BINGE EATING HABIT?

At the Core of the Matter

Although considerably more time and research has been dedicated to understanding bulimia nervosa and anorexia nervosa, scientific evidence is increasingly clear that as with these two eating disorders, three specific types of factors contribute to the binge-eating habit: biological, social, and psychological.

Genetically-speaking, like most psychological disorders, binge-eating patterns run in families. Although it is still unclear which biological determinants contribute to binge-eating (and other eating disorders), studies show that statistically, relatives of individuals with binge-eating disorder are 4 to 5 times more likely to develop the disorder than the general population (with female relatives a bit higher). It has been speculated that the unknown factor inherited through genetics may pertain to personality traits regarding emotional stability and impulse control. And while a number of more technical theories have been proposed (relating to specific areas of the brain and brain chemistry), the biological factor suggests that individuals may inherit a tendency to be emotionally reactive to life stressors, and as a consequence, respond to stressful events by eating impulsively in an attempt to reduce stress and anxiety.

Before this decade, anorexia nervosa and bulimia nervosa were the most rampant, culturally-specific psychological disorders yet known. Thousands of American middle- to upper-class teens were driven to self-punishing, life-threatening routines of starvation and/or purging as part of a cultural trend aimed at achieving super-thinness—the physical results pivotal to reaching unachievable levels of self-worth, happiness, and social acceptance. Shown to be directly related to TV and media exposure (teenage girls who watched 8 or more hours of TV per week reported significantly greater body dissatisfaction than those who watched less), body measurements alone came to dictate personal worth.

Similarly, America is again experiencing a distinct cultural trend, this time towards acceptance and promotion of larger body-types (particularly among people of Latin and African descent), reflected in the average breast size jumping from 34B to 34DD in less than two decades, and average butt size increasing from 41" to 45" (Black women averaging 46", Hispanic women, 44"), with breast and buttocks implants (to make these physical features more pronounced) growing in popularity. Thus, cultural trends continue to influence body image and eating habits to meet those trends.

Across the board, the psychological component of binge-eating (like other eating disorders) is by far the most consistent. While in some cases binge-eating behavior can be traced to a singularly traumatic event or organic cause, by and large, most binge-eaters suffer a marked diminished sense of self-control and confidence in their own abilities, manifested as critically low self-esteem, displayed as overt perfectionism. The binge-eating habit typically develops when perfectionism leads an individual to a distorted body image (often, body dysmorphism), as the individual attempts to create the "perfect" body—all the while having no confidence that they can actually achieve it. Their self-defeating mission is generally well under way by the time they decide to seek profession help, with biological and cultural components already embedded deep into the mindset.

So, what are the consequences if these biological and cultural components are left unaddressed?

CHAPTER 5: WHAT ARE THE HEALTH CONSEQUENCES OF BINGE EATING?

Considering the Binge-Eating-to-Obesity Pathway

Without question, binge-eating is serious—and not something to be taken lightly. For any man, woman, or child, the effects of this pernicious disorder can be absolutely devastating. In addition to the all-consuming emotional effects of binge-eating (guilt, shame, worthlessness, and depression), most binge-eaters suffer one or more of the following conditions: hyper-awareness, hormonal imbalances, hypertension, sleep disorders (especially insomnia, sleep apnea, and snoring), indigestion/gas and/or constipation, and any number of other conditions depending on the content of the binges-- tooth decay, skin rashes, and water retention, among many. And once this disorder transitions to obesity (as it commonly does when left untreated), the binge-eater is open to a whole new list of serious health concerns.

High blood pressure, osteoarthritis, reproductive problems in women (even affecting fertility), elevated cholesterol levels, coronary heart disease, stroke, Type II diabetes mellitus, and gallbladder disease are common among the obese. Additionally, recent studies have linked obesity to dementia and Alzheimer's disease (in later life), breast cancer (in postmenopausal women), neurological damage, and when left untreated, serious damage to internal organs. And just to drive home the seriousness of the binge-eating-to-obesity pathway, 1-in-5 American deaths are associated with obesity. And even if addressed before reaching the obesity stage, in that binge-eaters typically binge on huge quantities of foods that are high in fat, sugar, and/or salt and lack vitamins, minerals, and essential nutrients, even relatively short-term bingeing can result in malnutrition, the binge-eater suffering the effects of vitamin deficiency, including fatigue, dizziness, hair loss, and difficulty thinking.

Okay. So, what can be done?

CHAPTER 6: TREATMENT

Finding Your "Trigger"

At the core of every binge-eating habit lies a mystery to be solved: Why is binge-eating generally not a daily habit? Why is it that a binge-eater can go for several days eating regular, healthy meals then suddenly have the impulse to binge? Why is it that one day the bingeing habit seems under control and the next—it's not? The answer to these questions (and solving of this mystery) represents the first hurtle to treating this condition. Triggers.

Triggers are any sensory cue or stimulus that sets off unhealthy eating habits. A thought, an event, an environment, a circumstance, something—anything--that stimulates the senses and effectively turns on the bad-eating-habit "switch." For some, it's something obvious like the smell of pizza. Others, a recurring unpleasant memory that has no direct connection to food—but nonetheless sends the individual reaching for a box of cookies in an effort to escape it. And for others, it may be encountering a particular individual, place, or set of circumstances that suddenly makes food foremost in their minds.

But for some, the trigger is far more elusive. Seemingly undefined or constantly changing. Something that sneaks in and turns on the bad-eating-habit "switch" so stealthily that it leaves no trace—only the damage left in its wake. For most of those individuals, one of several psychological memory-retrieval therapies can expose that trigger to the light.

Drug Therapy

Among the various therapy options available to the binge-eater are a number of drugs found to be effective in dealing with the symptoms of binge-eating (measured primarily by a reduction in the frequency of binge-eating episodes). Although to date no drug has proved singularly effective in treating binge-eating disorder (BED) specifically. As all eating disorders are born of a similar biological/cultural/psychological mindset and typically respond to antidepressant medications aimed at mood and anxiety disorders.

Psychologists often prescribe antidepressants as a preliminary step—even if the patient's "trigger" has yet to be identified. And while not a long-term solution, the use of antidepressant medications can keep the disorder from escalating in frequency, provide the sufferer a sense of empowerment (which can help in identifying their trigger), and in some cases, has been shown to enhance the effects of psychological treatment. In any case, it should be understood that current drug therapy can only address the symptoms—not the root cause.

Self-Help Group Therapy

Although the positive effects of group therapy are less easy to measure regarding binge-eaters specifically, some eating disorder suffers seem to respond particularly well to the support-group setting. Though no substitute for straight-forward psychological therapy, support groups can provide certain individuals a number of benefits including: alleviating anxiety (relating to feeling alone), improving coping skills, greater acceptance of their illness, decreased levels of worry, increased levels of optimism, improved daily functioning, and improved symptom management.

Of two general types potentially beneficial to individuals suffering eating disorders—those geared to general mental health, those geared specifically to eating disorders--participation in self-help groups for mental health can encourage more focused use of professional therapy, making the time invested more effective. And while self-help groups can improve self-esteem, accelerate recovery, improve decision-making skills, increase the ability to resist triggers (once identified), and improve social functioning, they have limited effect on reducing psychological symptoms related to binge-eating disorder (BED).

However, it should be noted that the endorsement of self-help group therapy by mainstream psychologists is not necessarily an endorsement of online self-help groups. In that successful treatment of binge-eating disorder for many individuals (as with bulimia and anorexia) is a matter of first stepping out of their comfort zone and actively seeking and committing to formal therapy, the remote nature of online groups effectively promotes isolation and sedentary behavior—making them far less effective than on-site groups, and could potentially hinder progress.

Psychological Therapy

Provided in a variety of styles and perspectives, psychological therapy (or psychotherapy) is typically practiced in a one-on-one clinical setting (with group therapy an option for follow-up or aftercare). While a number of therapeutic methods are in common practice (depending on the psychologist's own training), the general goal is to target eating behavior and associated attitudes pertaining to the overpowering importance and significant of body image (weight and shape) in that individual. And while some psychologists specialize in one particular approach, such as cognitive-behavioral therapy (the identification of unhealthy thoughts that trigger binge-eating behavior and replacing them with positive thoughts that promote healthy behavior), interpersonal therapy (which focuses on how personal relationships relate to one's tendency to binge), and dialectical therapy (that focuses on learning how to regulate emotions and stress), some of the more successful binge-eating disorder (BED) specialists use a multi-pronged approach: essentially trying a number of treatments until one shows effectiveness—joining elements of several if necessary.

No matter the approach employed, the therapist is tasked with not only eliminating (or greatly reducing) the incidence of binge-eating and helping the individual find an optimal weight they can be happy with, they must also address the shame, low self-esteem, and self-imposed limitations underlying the disorder. And this may warrant the use of hypnosis, biofeedback, family therapy, or other supportive modalities.

Alternative Therapies: Meditation and Marijuana

Although the health benefits of meditation have been known in the West for decades now, only recently has a direct connection been made with treating binge-eating disorder (BED). According to a study conducted at Maharishi University in Iowa, meditation has proved to have a profound effect on stress levels, demonstrated by a marked decrease in the stress hormone, cortisol. After just a few weeks of regular meditation, practitioners typically find themselves less controlled by stress; they are better able to cope with daily stressors.

Many binge-eaters use food as a method to relax and

decrease perceived stress and anxiety, they find that when they use meditation to relax (reduce stress and anxiety) they no longer need to use food for that purpose. Additionally, long-term meditation creates an inner awareness of thoughts, reactiveness, emotions, behaviors, and compulsions--and the actions/reactions they precipitate. As one begins to cultivate an understanding of how their brain functions via meditation, most individuals find increased control over compulsions and aberrant behavior, and are able to exert greater self-control over their eating impulses.

Similarly, although binge-eating has long been directly associated with marijuana use (the so-called "munchies"), new studies geared to gauging the effects of marijuana on those suffering binge-eating disorder have made some very interesting—if not unexpected—discoveries. While dealing with the munchies is indeed an ongoing task for the average pot smoker, when some binge-eaters partake of marijuana, an odd phenomenon occurs: they lose the desire to eat. This is not to suggest that smoking marijuana has the opposite effect on binge-eater as it does individuals with normal eating habits, only that the sense of relaxation (reduced stress and anxiety) and introspection created by smoking marijuana allow some binge-eaters to resist the impulse to eat to excess. Although, the results of this and similar studies are not endorsed by the psychological community at large as yet, in states where medical marijuana has been legalized, this type of alternate therapy may be a reasonable consideration.

I admit...I need help! What do I do?

CHAPTER 7: WRITING YOUR OWN PERSONAL SUCCESS STORY

Reality Check

Okay, so now you've arrived at the place where you've resigned yourself to the hard, cold reality that you're a "binge-eater." Like millions of individuals around the country (tens of millions worldwide) you have binge-eating disorder (BED), a serious condition that if left untreated can have life-threatening consequences. So, it now falls upon you to take the first step towards fixing it, and you have a pretty good idea of what you're up against.

So, where do you begin? That's easy.

Begin with this simple reality check: BED is treatable! In fact, some statistics place the binge-eating disorder treatment success rate at over 60 percent! That means it's your job to do all you can to make yourself part of that statistic. To write your own personal success story.

Deciding to Overcome Binge Eating

Overcoming binge eating is not an easy task. To truly change your eating habits, you have to ensure you are highly motivated to do so. To make it easier, ask yourself why you should overcome binge eating and use those reasons to motivate yourself.

Your Reasons for Changing Your Eating Habits

There are endless reasons for changing your eating habits, because nothing good can come of overeating and the consequential weight gain. You can start reducing your binge eating habits at a slow and steady pace and go back to normal eating portions. Getting rid of this disorder will also help you ditch the guilt and shame.

Going back to regular eating habits will also mean you won't have to eat in secrecy anymore and life suddenly becomes more enjoyable. The anxieties that arise before binge eating will eventually go away and food will stop controlling your life. Soon enough, your emotional and physical health will start to improve and you will stop stressing over negative emotions. It's almost like flying out of a cage.

Whatever your reasons are, use those reasons to stay motivated because when the feeling to binge arises, you will need to stay strong. Recovery is almost impossible if there is a lack of motivation. To motivate yourself, make a list of things you will gain from continuing your binge eating habits and also if you stop binge eating.

Be as honest as you can about what you want for yourself, and soon enough, you will see that the balance is tipping in favor of the latter. Never force yourself towards change, only stay motivated.

You will also need a support system to get yourself through this drastic change. This can be a family, friend, or colleague. The type of support you need depends on your personal situation. Also, make sure you choose an appropriate time to bring these changes. If you are planning to go on holiday or are experiencing a rather stressful situation right now, maybe it's not a good time to start.

Lastly, make sure you are comfortable and ready to commit. Don't postpone it without a solid reason because you never know when your level of motivation will rise again. If you feel some motivation now, bank on it.

Measuring Success

Before you begin the recovery process, it's important to have a clear vision of your objective. Every binge-eater's success story can be likened to a long journey; a step-by-step quest that will have its uphill climbs and downhill runs—some legs more challenging than others. There will be rocky patches and obstacles--but also level ground and clear pathways. And like a long journey, the rewarding moments are not confined to reaching your destination, they are found around every bend, at every crossroads. Like mile-markers that file by as you make your way, so too will the mile-stones of progress—each one a significant step towards reaching your goal. This journey isn't measured by how quickly or directly you reach your destination—only that you do. For many, it's a matter of baby steps (one foot in front of the other). And for much of your journey, your mental-health therapist will be your guide.

Psychological Intervention

Although psychotherapy isn't usually regarded as "intervention," in a very real sense it is. When an individual with binge-eating disorder (BED) seeks the help of a psychologist, he/she is effectively asking the mental health specialist to intervene on their behalf. To get between them and their illness. And so it should be understood that in working with a psychotherapist to find a way to break the binge-eating habit, the individual must trust in that therapist's ability to do just that. To give themselves to the process and put themselves in their therapist's capable hands. Any resistance will invariably impede progress, and delay success.

As explained earlier, psychologists who specialize in treating eating disorders come from a variety of schools of thought—meaning a number of approaches and strategies are in common use. Some use straight-forward cognitive or behavioral therapy, while others routinely use a multi-leveled approach, having you consult with a nutritionist, medical doctor, clinical social worker, or other healthcare professional. Some work one-on-one exclusively--while others prefer a group or family setting. Accordingly, some approaches are much more intensive in nature than others.

No matter the approach, the goal of the therapist is to seek to discover the underlying factors of your binge-eating episodes (and prevent you from resisting the binge-eating impulse), monitor your episodes and change the way you react to your "triggers," while finding an inroad to restoring your self-image.

Most binge-eaters have reached a critical point of desperation before ever seeking professional help (trying but failing to control it on their own), the therapist must invariably untangle a complex web of mental and physical issues that serve to obscure the underlying issue.

Admittedly, this is a highly interpersonal process that can be quite slow-going. But every new insight—every new element of self-discovery--brings you one step closer to regaining control of your life. It goes without saying that patience is essential to recovery and that each mile-stone should be seen as a significant step forward.

Regarding Sex and Age Factors

While there are at least 20 psychotherapeutic approaches to treating eating disorders in use today (all of which may be used exclusively or in tandem with other therapies in treating binge-eating disorder), varying levels of effectiveness have been noted with regards to sex and age. For example, the feminist psychodynamic therapy model (based on the premise that social conditioning of women results in the repression of certain needs) appears to be especially effective with women coming from urban settings. Similarly, the family therapy model(s) (which typically provide treatment for both patient and family) is often more effective in treating adolescents still living at home. But unlike the former demographics, men seem to respond better to gender/sex-specific, professionally-led eating disorder support groups; obese men seeming to respond to the cognitive-behavioral group therapy model (which focuses on triggers, behaviors, and consequences of binge-eating).

CHAPTER 8: TEN EFFECTIVE REINFORCEMENT STRATEGIES

Positive Reinforcement Dos and Don'ts

Whether you're in the beginning or latter stages of recovering your self-control, there are a number of valuable strategies (dos and don'ts) that can help speed up the process or lend support to the progress you've already made. For example:

- Do Eat Breakfast Every Morning. Whether eating breakfast comes naturally to you or not, starting your day with something substantial in your stomach (and not just coffee and a bagel) can help keep the urges at bay throughout the day. Statistically, individuals who skip breakfast weigh more and are more vulnerable to evening-hour bingeing.
- Do Drink Water Religiously. The essential nature of water for the body cannot be overstated. In addition to the dozens of bodily process it makes possible, water serves to break down and distribute the contents of food, making so-called cravings less powerful.
- Do Establish a Regular Sleep Routine. Numerous

studies have shown that individuals who are able to establish a regular sleep and eating routine (going to bed at a regular time, eating breakfast in the morning soon after waking, with lunch and dinner also at regular times) are less responsive to binge triggers.

- Do Learn to Take Walks. Although walking is often associated with "working up an appetite," the meditative aspects of daily strolls (aided by endorphins secreted) have been shown to have a profound effect on mood and outlook. Binge-eaters who have adopted regular walking habits report reduced stress, better sleep, and subsequently, better resistance to food triggers.

- Do Keep a Diary. One of the most effective tools an individual can utilize when going through any challenging time, a diary lets you acknowledge your trials and successes, as well as note personal discoveries regarding your disorder—both positive and negative. (Expect your therapist to suggest this.)

- Do Not Compensate for Bad Eating Habits with Fast-Food "Healthy Menus." Despite what appears to be an effort on the part of the fast-food industry to provide the public with healthy food options, the fact is, these so-called healthy choices contain deceptive amounts of sugar, salt, and preservatives that can drastically alter blood and brain chemistry. Rather than satiate hunger, these additives are designed to stimulate hunger—which can send binge-eaters into an eating frenzy.

- Do Not Eat Processed Foods. While avoiding junk- and fast-food may be a no-brainer for most, it's important to understand that processed foods (prepackaged, dried, frozen, canned) contain the same unhealthy chemicals that make junk- and fast-food dangerous. In fact, tossing out all processed foods from the cupboards, pantry, and refrigerator should be one of the first steps the recovering binge-eater takes.

- Do Not Diet. Unless your therapist has suggested a particular dietary plan as part of the psychotherapeutic process, do not begin a diet during the recovery process. Most diets make substantive biochemical changes in the body that can interfere with the recovery process, and even cause a set-back.

- Do Not Live like a Hermit. Even though you may see your binge-eating triggers as the "enemies," you cannot go through life isolating yourself to avoid them. Ultimately, it's the desensitization of your triggers that empower you and allow you to live a normal life. And the only way to make that possible is to expose yourself to environments where those triggers exist.

- Do Not Lie to Yourself. Whether you prefer the personal mantra "to thine own self be true" or "keep it real," the principle is extremely important to your success. Never, ever lie to yourself about your progress or your set-backs. Part of the recovery process is learning to trust yourself. And truth is the foundation of trust.

Watching Your Food Intake

The first step to changing your eating habits is to watch your current food intake. Simply start recording everything you eat and drink, including how you feel when you are eating. Do you feel like you ate too much? Did you feel out of control? Record all the relevant details.

Initially, you might find it hard to record everything because it's almost as if you are confronting your eating disorder. It's like the walk of shame when writing down what and how much you ate after a binge.

However, if you really want to bring change, you must start putting it down in pen and paper to truly realize how much you are consuming. Don't feel de-motivated because recording your food intake is the first step towards making a change for the better.

When recording your daily food intake, use a simple form because anything too complicated will make the process harder for no reason. Use a separate sheet for each day. Record everything, including things that made you feel guilty or sad. Record right away so you don't miss anything.

After you have recorded your food intake for about a week or so, go back and review what you ate. See if there are any patterns that will help you figure out your binge eating triggers. Use this data to find valuable information so you can come up with techniques to start regaining control of your eating habits.

When you are reviewing your eating records, reflect on how honest you have been when you wrote it down. If you did modify something, ask yourself why? If you are changing your records so they feel more "acceptable", those feelings could be further explored to start the recovery process.

Creating a Meal Plan

The best way to reduce cravings and overcome binging is by eating regularly and not staying hungry for longer than 3 hours. When you stay hungry for long periods of time in hopes of losing weight, your metabolism goes berserk.

Your body's metabolism is the rate at which the food is converted into energy. Restricting your food intake or bingeing can really mess up your metabolism. When you decrease food intake, your body starts to conserve energy and the metabolic rate drops. Bingeing, on the other hand, increases your metabolic rate because there is so much food that needs to be converted into energy.

Eating every 2 to 3 hours will take you out of your binge eating cycle. When you know you will be eating again in a couple of hours, it will help you calm down and reduce your urge to binge. If you are tempted to binge, remind yourself of your next scheduled meal so you can finally escape the vicious cycle.

When creating your meal plan, you will still have breakfast, lunch and dinner, with two snack times. During this routine, stay mindful of the fact that you are not trying to restrict your diet or eat large portions. This new eating pattern is just right and will help you enter the recovery process.

Continue recording your meals even after you have implemented the new meal plan. This will help you realize if the newly devised diet is working or not. If you do happen to binge, make sure you record that as well. Later, when you are reviewing your records, try to figure out what triggered the binge so you can avoid it down the road.

Incorporating Healthy Eating Habits

Your new eating habits should be treated as a change, not as a diet. Diets have a negative connotation to them, and you end up associating it with frustration and a feeling of being trapped. Your newly changed eating habits are not about the right diet, but about developing your sense of self where food and weight are not correlated. Choose foods that are satisfying so you are able to make the changes in a comfortable manner. Depriving yourself of your favorite foods may trigger your binge eating habits.

At first, it might be difficult to switch to low-calorie food, but as long as you are getting enough to eat, you should do well. Stay mindful of the fact that you are not trying to control your weight. Instead, you are trying to improve your health. When health becomes priority, food choices become much easier.

Your energy levels and mood also depend on the type of food you eat. To figure out what foods help you feel better, refer to your food diary. This way, you can make changes that will improve your overall eating habits. If you are unable to figure out patterns or triggers that make you binge, consult a dietitian. Use your food diary to help figure out the problem. You never know what type of complex problem you could be dealing with, such as irregular blood sugar levels.

Plan and prepare your meals in advance so you can control your portions. In most restaurants, the menus will have "starters", but in your case, you need an "ender". End your meals with a piece of fruit or bread so you know your meal has ended and you cannot eat any more.

Preparing your food in advance will also help you make more mindful choices and you will be less inclined to overstock foods. To make things easier for yourself, don't shop for a whole week, but rather practice control by shopping for two to three days.

Initially, you will be responding to your natural hunger, but soon enough you will fall in with your scheduled meal plan. Be mindful of triggers and avoid them at all costs, such as being alone on the weekend. If you eat out of boredom, for instance, plan an activity for yourself, such as a DIY project.

Spending unstructured time will definitely trigger a binge, especially if you are on holiday. For that reason, always keep yourself busy so you can cope with your eating disorder. Whenever you finish eating, you should have a feeling of comfort and satisfaction, the lack of which could cause you to binge. Take your time in tasting the food instead of gulping it down. The more you enjoy your food, the more satisfied you will be.

Try to avoid alcohol as you make changes to your eating habits because it's a common trigger. A lot of people find it hard to control their eating after drinking alcohol and the consequential hangover could also trigger binge eating.

When you plan your meals, you might find yourself thinking about food all the time, but don't let it stress you out. This is normal and only happens for a short while till you get accustomed to the new routine. Make sure you stick to the eating choices you have planned in advance.

Also, consider your energy expenditure. If your activity levels were relatively high, maybe snack time can happen an hour earlier, and if not, consider skipping that snack altogether. If you constantly feel hungry after a meal, you might need to review your meal plan.

When you are changing your eating habits, it might not always be supported by the people around you. For that reason, let everyone know about your change in eating habits so you are not gifted a box of chocolates or treats. If you have kids, you might feel it's really difficult to manage a healthy eating meal plan with them, but it could instead be an opportunity to introduce them to healthy eating as well.

Keep things flexible so your newly devised meal plan remains strong. Rigidity will not help you go for long. There is no reason for your entire family to follow the same meal plan as yours. If you all eat the same food, you won't feel like you are on a diet. This will also make meal planning fairly easy because a last minute binge won't change the menu. It will also hold you accountable to the rest of your family members so you are less likely to fail.

Stop Dieting

Dieting is one of the major precipitating factors for someone suffering from binge eating disorder. However, it also plays a big role in maintaining your eating disorder. Trying to figure out the underlying reasons behind your eating disorder is a tough task and that is why you find yourself in a vicious cycle of binge eating and dieting.

So, break the cycle by stopping your crazy diet. It may be a little unsettling as you feel like you have lost control on your binge, but try to reflect on how the diet affects your lifestyle. When you realize that dieting is promoting your eating disorder, it will be easier to let go of it.

When you steadily replace your binge eating and dieting habits with a well-planned meal schedule, it is unlikely for you to gain weight. If you feel your body is not experiencing any change, don't panic. Change doesn't happen overnight and it takes a long time to unwind all the binge eating sessions. However, the silver lining is that soon enough, the needle on the weighing scale will start sliding back and you will become a better version of you.

Your food diary should now be able to show you patterns where you have been either binge eating or dieting. For the next few weeks, consider situations where you restricted yourself from eating, reached out for comfort food, felt guilty about eating, or had the urge to diet again.

By understanding your feelings about dieting and binge eating, you will make it easier on yourself. If that's too hard, try sharing your feelings with someone who understands what you are going through.

Often, the fear of getting fat will prevent the person from giving up on the diet. You could look at this from another perspective. Stop dieting for a while, at least for a few weeks or so. Follow your devised meal plan and keep recording your food intake.

During this diet, watch out for any improvement and identify factors that have been triggering your eating disorders. At times, you might feel physically bigger, which could urge you to restrict food. This is the time to stay strong because otherwise, you will fall into the vicious cycle all over again. Merely stopping the diet for a few days could possibly break the cycle forever.

CHAPTER 9: RELAPSE PREVENTION

Changing the Way, You Think

Your desire to eat shapes your body weight and your feelings towards it. You can stop dieting by changing your eating habits and if you want your eating behaviors to last forever, it is important to challenge your thoughts and feelings as well.

The way you think and feel about yourself can have a significant impact on everything you do. The way you feel about yourself is directly reflective in your weight and shape, which in turn, decides your eating habits. Losing weight will obviously make you feel you are a better person and gaining weight will make you feel as if you have failed yourself.

You also become more conscious of the way other people think about you. The reality is that none of these feelings actually represents the truth. You remain the same person you are, regardless of your weight and shape, and the people around you think of you the same way as well.

A major part of recovery is to start building a more positive image of yourself by changing your thought patterns. You can do this by first cutting yourself some slack and minimizing self-criticism. If you find yourself making negative comments about yourself, shut it down. Come up with a strategy that turns all your negative thoughts into positive thoughts.

A good way is to challenge all your negative thoughts, for instance, "I look so fat in this dress, but I still look pretty and it makes me comfortable." Alternatively, whenever you find yourself criticizing, stop and compliment yourself instead. As soon as you start treating yourself better, you will eventually build a better view of your body, which will translate into better eating habits as well. Remember that the way you think is directly reflective on your physical health.

Coping with Difficult Emotions

Binge eating is often triggered by uncomfortable feelings. When you eat, you might find a temporary sense of relief as your feelings are zoned out and your problems come to a halt, at least until you are eating. To tackle this type of binge eating, you need to face your emotions head-on to truly start the recovery process.

It might require you to admit these feelings to a colleague, discuss unpleasant issues with your partner, or maybe wrinkle out problems with your child. Whatever situation you are dealing with has to be resolved rather than avoided. Naming it what it is will help you deal with it so you can finally move on and relieve your urge to binge.

To find out your triggers for binge eating, look for thoughts or feelings that make you feel upset. Then decide for yourself if those feelings are rational or irrational. If you cannot find a direct solution for the problem, the feelings are most likely irrational, such as feelings of hate towards oneself due to body shape. In that case, start making your thoughts more rational, such as stressing over body shape is of no use, but exercising is.

Reflecting on Body Image

When you build positive feelings about your body shape and size, it starts to increase confidence in your body shape. Valuing yourself as you are will allow you to enjoy life without having to worry about dieting or losing weight. Feeling confident about your body will help you see food as part of healthy living, instead of a coping mechanism. You will start to develop a sense of "good" foods and "bad" foods. Here are a few ways you can improve your body image.

You need to look beyond just the physical aspects of yourself. You are much more than meat and bones. Focus less on your appearance and more on yourself as a whole person who has other qualities.

- Define the meaning of being healthy. Being healthy means you should be well rested, well fed, at ease and thinking clearly. You should be feeling good about yourself, inside and out.
- Give yourself a pep talk and use a mirror if it helps. Remind yourself of the qualities you like about yourself and what you would like others to appreciate. Believe in yourself!
- Tell yourself that you do not need to be like anyone else and you are who you are. Telling yourself to be like someone else is like an apple wanting to be an orange. Everybody is different and has different body shapes. You need to learn to accept your uniqueness, instead of trying to be someone you are not. Celebrate your differences and do not grieve for them.
- Take risks by challenging yourself. Do something that you would not normally do, for instance, spend a day at the spa or go swimming. Taking care of yourself and spending some leisure time will help you recover faster.
- Go somewhere by yourself, somewhere where you can

bring your thoughts together and get to know yourself. You should be the first person you love.

- Focus on your qualities and talents that make you proud. You do not have to be hard on yourself all the time. However, do not ignore qualities you do not like about yourself either. Come up with ways to change them in a positive manner. If you feel you are overweight, start an exercise routine. If you feel like you are socially awkward, then attend places where you can socialize. If you do not like your job, start looking for a new one. Do whatever it takes to fix the unhappy aspects of your life.

One Step Forward, Two Steps Back

A word no one wants to hear in the treatment of eating disorders, "relapse" is defined as the reappearance of an eating disorder symptom, or the deterioration of an individual's condition, following the initially successful response to treatment. And as regards binge-eating disorder (BED), there is good news and bad regarding this state. The bad news, of course, is that it happens all too often. It can be disheartening and exasperating. The good news, however, is that in fact, it's likely to happen—and more than once. Which makes it a normal part of the recovery process! And as such, a great deal of concerted study has gone into understanding what it means when a patient essentially "takes two steps back." And most psychologists agree that in most cases, the less made of it, the better. A relapse is not a sign of failure, but simply an indicator that there is more work to be done. Even so, there are a number of behaviors that can signal that a relapse is likely:

For one, a sudden increase in obsessive thinking about food and/or weight. For another, feelings of self-doubt preventing an individual from eating even normal amounts of food. Skipping meals, daily weigh-ins, and self-inspections in the mirror may also be signals.

Likewise, a resurgence of perfectionist attitudes, withdrawal from friends and/or family, and any significant change in outward appearance may forewarn that a relapse is on the horizon. But even if these behaviors present themselves, keep in mind that there may be little that can be done to prevent a full-blown relapse from occurring, and only makes a difference in the recovery process if it's allowed to. When the crisis passes, the best thing the individual can do is simply pick up from where they left off in the recovery process. Pick up and move forward towards the goal without hesitation.

CHAPTER 10: TAKING CARE OF YOURSELF

Maintaining Your Physical Health

If you suffer from binge eating disorder, chances are you are not completely satisfied with your body. People who are not fond of their physique usually consider themselves separate from their bodies. They avoid looking at themselves in the mirror, touching themselves or even letting anyone else get physically close to them.

When you do not like your body, you tend to stop caring for it. To start loving your body again, there are many small things you can do. For instance, you can get a massage, a haircut or even a new perfume to just feel more connected to your body.

You can further improve feelings about your body with exercise. Exercise offers more benefits than just weight management. It increases your metabolism and puts your body in a healthy routine. Regular exercising prevents many chronic diseases and the high levels of activity keep you focused as well. However, the best part about exercise is that it makes an excellent coping mechanism for stress, which in turn can help you overcome your desire to binge.

Regular exercise requires a high level of commitment, but as soon as you bring it into routine, it will get easier every day. In fact, people who start exercising regularly feel amiss even with one missed exercise session. Of course, in the beginning you will need to boost your motivation because things like weather or other circumstances could become an excuse to skip exercise.

Maintaining Your Emotional Health

To recover from an eating disorder, it's important to develop a holistic approach to mind and body. You have to start acknowledging the fact that your mind and body are connected and are not separate entities. For that reason, you need to start taking care of the emotional side of you. Learn to face your emotions on a regular basis instead of burying them inside. Here are a few ways you can enhance your health by addressing your emotions:

Recognize the emotion by giving it a name, be it anger, despair, sadness or regret. If you are facing an extremely difficult situation, it might be helpful to think in a quiet place to truly identify your feelings.

- Identify the emotion in your body and give it all your attention. Simply sit down and start taking deep breaths. Allow yourself to become fully aware of all your physical sensations and keep going until all you feel is the emotion. This will help you recognize your feelings and you will start seeing how your feelings are affecting you as a person.
- Your feelings are nobody's fault and for that reason, you have to take responsibility for your feelings. However, don't think that what you are feeling is either justified or unjustified. Often, you will experience a wide range of emotions in a short period of time, and there doesn't need to be a whole lot of

reasons for it. All you need to do is understand those feelings and find the right reaction for it.

For instance, when someone asks you to do something when you're already under pressure, you might be inclined to not do it, or even lash out in anger, though, in reality, all you needed to do was say 'no'. By truly understanding your feelings, you can escape the emotional turmoil and find appropriate solutions. When you know you have the power to choose and stay in control, you are more likely to make better decisions. At the end of the day, you are only responsible for your own feelings, not everyone else's.

- You also need to express your feelings, either to yourself or someone you trust. Merely saying it out loud will make you feel a whole lot better. You can even write it down and outline specific details relative to how you are feeling. This is a strong way of releasing all your built-up emotions.
- Lastly, treat yourself to something that makes you happy.

Handling Difficult Situations

On your path to recovery, you will experience days when it will be difficult to resist the urge to binge. However, don't let a small setback or slip let you abandon your meal plan and continue bingeing. Set things straight right away and do it as soon as possible. The more you delve into your temptations, the harder it will be to get back on track.

Just stop and think about what you are doing. If you need to step out of the house and take a breather, do so. This is also a good time to contact your support system, whoever it may be. Use their words of encouragement to help you stay strong. Whenever you slip, remember it is in your power to put an end to it.

So, as soon as you had your small slip, get back to your eating plan as soon as possible. Ignore all excuses that your brain might come up with and never skip a meal to make up for your binge. Continue with your meal plan as scheduled. It can be difficult to keep going because you just overate and you will have a strong temptation to stay hungry, but going back to the meal plan will prevent you from having another episode where you lose control.

What you can do is instead of having a full meal, eat something light. Of course, that doesn't mean that you eat an apple. Have a complete meal. If your small setback has overwhelmed you with fear, anxiety or feelings of self-disgust, seek your support system right away. This is the time you face your feelings and come out stronger. Remember that these feelings are normal and all you have to do is look beyond it and return to your path of recovery.

Do your best to avoid feeling disappointed with yourself or let a small setback make you feel like you have failed. Everyone makes mistakes and instead of abandoning your months of effort, simply learn from your mistake. Use that mistake to avoid future mistakes because it's all part of your personal evolvement. Try to see it as a simple fact and reserve judgment.

Not judging yourself is another skill you have to develop in order to maintain a positive attitude about yourself. It's one of the best things you can do to boost your self-esteem. Slips and setbacks are part of the recovery process and all you need to do is treat it as a learning experience.

Look at the things that went wrong. Did you eat enough at your previous meal? Was it triggered by an event or feeling? Reflecting back on your setback will allow you to avoid it in the future. Talking to someone can be really helpful at this point because often you are oblivious to your own actions. A person seeing your situation from a different angle may be better able to pinpoint why your binge eating disorder got triggered.

If this is not the first time that you have had a setback, think back to the last time you slipped and how you recovered from it. Maybe you can use the same method to recover again. Also, look at your setbacks in a positive manner so you know how to move forward from this. Let your setback become a motivating factor for you instead of letting yourself feel stressed and defeated.

Think of it this way: you are striving to reduce the number of times you binge, instead of trying to never binge again. This makes your small setbacks an achievement, because before that, you binged all the time. Remember, you are not back to square one, but simply at a place where the bingeing has considerably decreased. You were successful before; you can do it again.

CHAPTER 11: FINAL THOUGHTS

Prognosis

The prevalence of binge-eating disorder (BED) in the U.S. and around the world has made this all-too common disease one of the most studied among members of the medical and psychological communities--particularly with its direct connection to sky-rocketing obesity numbers in the U.S. (and elsewhere), and incidence of compulsive eating disorder (CED) and anorexia nervosa binge-eating/purging (AN-BP). And while no one form of therapy has to date proved superior in treating BED, this appears to merely reflect the individual nature of binge-eating disorder sufferers; symptoms are as individual as the personality behind them. Still, as our understanding of this pernicious disease grows, so too does the recovery rate—which is already encouragingly high. Bottom line: This disease is treatable. And with the right dedication, you too can free yourself of its hold.

RESOURCES

Ahrberg, M., D. Trojca, N. Nasrawi, and S. Vocks. (2011). "Body Image Disturbances in Binge-Eating Disorder: A Review." Accessed via: Wiley Online Library, DOI: 10.1002/ erv. 1100

American Psychiatric Association website. (2013). Diagnostic and Statistical Manual of Mental Disorders, (5th ed). Accessed via: dsm.psychiatryonline.org

BEDA (Binge Eating Disorder Association) website: http://bedaonline.com/understanding-binge-eating-disorder/

Durand, M. and D. Barlow (2012). Essentials of Abnormal Psychology. CA: Thomson Wadsworth.

EDC (Eating Disorders Coalition) website: http://eatingdisorderscoalition.org/

Hallett, C. and J. Kristeller. "An Exploratory Study of a Meditation-Based Intervention for Binge- Eating Disorder." Journal of Health Psychology. Accessed via: http://hpq.sagepub.com/content/4/3/357.short

Heatherton, T. and R. Baumeister. (July 1991). "Binge-Eating as Escape from Self-Awareness."

Psychological Bulletin, Vol 110(1).

International Journal of Eating Disorders. (April 1992). "Binge-Eating Disorder: A Multi-Site Field Trial of the Diagnostic Criteria." Volume 11, Issue 3.

Judd, S., ed. (2011). Eating Disorders Sourcebook. MI: Omnigraphics, Inc.

Kittleson, M., ed. (2004). "The Truth About Eating Disorders." New York: Facts on File.

Lefton, L. Psychology. Boston: Allyn and Bacon.

Mayo Clinic website: "Binge-Dating Disorder." Accessed via: http://www.mayoclinic.org/diseases-conditions/binge-eating-disorder/home/ovc-20182926

Mazzeo, S. (January 2009). "Environmental and Genetic Risk Factors for Eating Disorders: What the Clinician Needs to Know." Accessed via: US National Library of Medicine National Institutes of Health website: https://www.ncbi.nlm.nih.gov/pmc/articles/PMC271956 1/

NIH (National Institutes of Health) website: http://www.niddk.nih.gov/health-information/health-statistics/Pages/overweight-obesity-statistics.aspx

People's Daily Online website. "Binge Eating Affects Large Number of Americans: A Survey." Accessed via: http://en.people.cn/200702/05/print20070205_347678.h tml

ABOUT THE AUTHOR

Edward Standmore is a reader, an author and an entrepreneur with a passion to put research into the hands of the everyday person, so you can fulfill your goals.

Edward has experienced many problems, heartaches and disappointments and he wants to help you overcome your problems and find true happiness.

Sometimes people need a little help on their happiness journey.

Edward can help you reach your destination.